# GMO Free Diet

## *The Ultimate Guide on Avoiding GMO Foods and keeping Your Family Healthy with a GMO Free Diet*

# Table of Contents

The information herein is offered for informational purposes solely, and is universal as so. The presentation of the information is without contract or any type of guarantee assurance.

The trademarks that are used are without any consent, and the publication of the trademark is without permission or backing by the trademark owner. All trademarks and brands within this book are for clarifying purposes only and are the owned by the owners themselves, not affiliated with this document.

# Introduction

**I want to thank you and congratulate you for downloading the book, "*GMO Free Diet: The ultimate Guide on avoiding GMO foods and keeping your family healthy with a GMO Free Diet*"**

This book contains proven steps and strategies on how you can finally say *adieu* to a diet filled with potentially harmful organisms and ingredients. The book itself is a good educational tool that you can use to disarm your lifestyle with the unnecessary use and intake of GMOs.

Furthermore, the book leads you towards your ultimate goal – keeping you, and your family healthy. There is a wealth of knowledge contained in this book. To give you a glimpse, here are a few valuable highlights you will benefit from:

#1: You will understand how GMOs react once they reach your digestive tract. Trust me, it is NOT GOOD!

#2: You will finally decode those hard-to-read ingredients in the labels of your favorite cereals, canned foods, sweets, etc.

#3: You will start embracing a new lifestyle that is healthier and worth all the hard work. Now, that's enticing!

So before I start spilling all the beans here, you can start discovering the entire truth about GMOs with every flip of the page.

Thanks again for downloading this book, I hope you enjoy it!

# Chapter 1- GMOs: The Big No-No!

Genetically Modified Organisms (or GMOs) have swept the world of consumption and biotechnology industry in a very controversial manner. The term itself has prompted several countries to ban their production. Many skeptical consumers have likewise challenged state laws in making GMO labeling mandatory in all food products sold on the market.

*BUT the question is – what really are these so-called GMOs?*

To quote World Health Organization's definition: "GMOs are organisms in which the genetic material (DNA) has been altered in a way that does not occur naturally".

As the name suggests, GMOs are 'genetically engineered' foods or crops. The genetic makeup of these foods is modified or manipulated artificially through validated genetic engineering process. The process has created a range of produce, which are engineered so as to control characteristics such as disease resistance, pesticide resistance, herbicide resistance, nutritional content, and even ripening. Thus, this is a new science that evidently produces 'unstable' bacteria and viruses that could never be produced through natural methods. To put simply, GMOs are 'manipulated' to confer certain traits that are not natural for the organism.

Commercial GMOs have anchored their way on the global market through enticing promises which include:

- Increased yield

- Climate-change ready crops

- Reduced need for the use of pesticides and/or herbicides

- Improved nutrition content of the crops compared to naturally grown produce

- Reduced risks of food shortage

On the other hand, with the growing popularity of GMOs come a range of issues connected to environmental damages and health problems, as well as the violation of farmers' rights and consumer's rights.

**So how did GMOs break into the global market?**

The transfer of DNA from one organism to another was found possible and viable back in 1946. However, the real application took place roughly four decades after this discovery. The first ever recorded genetically modified/engineered plant came about in 1983, when a tobacco plant was made anti-biotic resistant.

In 1994, The Food and Drug Administration in the US approved the sale of 'Flavr Savr' tomato, the first food-related genetically modified organism. The company, Calgene in California, started to produce this tomato variant using genetically engineered seeds that have been injected with ACC synthase. Such gene allows ripening to take place after the tomatoes have been picked manually. This particular product has also become a catalyst for the production of more GMOs- particularly the BT corn, BT potato, and canola. Glyphosate (herbicide) –resistant squash followed suit. In 2010, another GMO breakthrough was recorded when scientists were able to augment the Vitamin A content of rice. This rice variant has been on the commercial market ever since.

# Chapter 2- Busting the GMO Myths

**Myth #01**: GMOs increase the yield potential of the crop

**Truth #01**: GMOs DO NOT increase yield potential, they may even decrease yield potential of the crop.

High yield is regarded as a complex genetic potential that is based on multi-faceted genetic function. Therefore, increased yield can never be genetically engineered in any crop. Data obtained by earthopensource.org show that the non-GMO agricultural productivity in Western Europe is much better than the GMO productivity in the US. Agroecological practices and conventional breeding are still considered two of the top reasons for productive agricultural yields.

The US Department of Agricultural has released a report that contradicts this particular myth. According to a USDA report of 2002, 'commercially available, genetically modified crops do not show increase yield potential.' Another report in 2014 stated GE (genetically engineered) has not shown any augmentation in yield potentials. Moreover, the herbicide-tolerant seeds may offer lower yields if they contain BT or HT genes."

**Myth #02:** GMOs are climate change-ready.

**Truth #02:** Climate change resistance does not solely depend on plant genetics

GMO producers have claimed again and again that crops, which are genetically modified can withstand any severe weather conditions. However, this is completely false as weather resistance of crops highly depends on the complex and invariable genetic traits. Moreover, conventional breeding of crops is still way far ahead than genetic engineering when it comes to delivering crops that are truly climate-ready. Tolerance to climate change partly lies in agroecological techniques widely used today. Some commonly used techniques to prepare crops in extreme weather situations include diversity crop planting and soil building.

**Myth #03**: GMOs can help farmers reduce the use of pesticides/herbicides

**Truth #03**: GMOs prompt the use of more pesticides/herbicides

GMO producers have claimed that the production of GMO crops decreases the use of pesticides. However, this is completely untrue. Herbicide-tolerant GMOs make use of a significant amount of glyphosate-based chemicals (e.g. Roundup), which technically is a herbicide. In other words, the reduced pesticide used is replaced by a massive use of herbicide. Consequently, the growing cultivation of herbicide-tolerant crops has led to the production of 'superweeds'. This so-called 'chemical treadmill' in farming has been proven unsustainable and questionable, particularly for farmers in the southern hemisphere.

**Myth #04:** GMOs improve the nutrition content of the crops compared to naturally bred produce

**Truth #04:** GMOs have manifested nutritional side-effects caused by genetic alteration

"Healthier and far more nutritional value in agricultural crops" is the promise of GMO producers. However, there are still no nutritionally enhanced, genetically modified products available in the market. Moreover, due to the miscalculated effects caused by genetic engineering, there are now studies proving that GMO products are far less nutritious than their naturally grown counterparts. 'Biofortified' crops, such as the GM Golden Rice, are still not readily available in the market due to the ongoing toxicological testing.

**Myth #05:** GMOs can help reduce the risks of food shortage

**Truth #05:** Food security can only be achieved through agroecological farming

The International Assessment of Agricultural Knowledge, Science and Technology for Development (IAASTD) report in 2008, which was highly supported by 58 countries, points out that GM crops are not the key to food security. Moreover, the report highlights that GMOs cannot be endorsed due to safety concerns, inconsistent yields, and restrictive seed patents. The report also expressed that food security can be achieved through the agroecological system of food production. This report was based on a four-year project sponsored by World Bank and carried out by 400 scientists from 80 different countries.

8

# Chapter 3 – 10 Reasons to Say NO to GMO

Food is vital to the survival – this is one fact that no one can contest. However, the type of food we eat makes the 'survival', *err*, relative. The consumption of GMOs has been contested by many countries and a hundred other organizations due to one major concern – SAFETY.

Technically speaking, the potential causes of the health hazards from GMO food consumption can be summarized in three points:

1.  Certain GMO products (e.g. Bt toxin found in insecticidal products) may be highly allergenic;

2.  The genetic alteration may lead to mutagenic effects that can disturb the normal processes of the biological structure;

3.  Toxic residues may be produced due to changes in farming practices.

Following is a set of studies conducted with GMO foods being fed to rats and rabbits resulting in adverse health effects, giving you hopefully a big reason why you should say NO to GMO:

**Reason #1: Multiple organ damage and failure, male fertility effects and modified blood biochemistry**

One study comparing the impact of GMO food to non-GMO food showed that rats, which were fed with Ajeeb YG (A Monsanto variant) experienced massive changes in body weight as well as changes in the fatty degeneration in the liver. Other abnormalities found included excessive growth and death of villi, blood vessel congestion in the kidneys, and desquamation of the spermatogonial cells.

**Reason #2: Disturbances in the Immunity**

Mice of various ages were fed with GMO Bt Maize for a month-long period. The impact showed a significant disturbance within their biochemical activity and cells in charge of the immune system. To be more specific, there were inflammatory responses observed due to the serum cytokines poisoning.

**Reason #3:  Allergic reaction and adverse immune responses**

Mice which were fed with alpha-amylase inhibitor (insecticidal protein) sustained a strong immunity against GM protein. Antibodies were developed, which allowed the hypersensitivity reaction to delay. This means that the insecticidal protein acts as a sensitizer, which made the mice more susceptible to developing allergies as compared to consuming non-allergenic type of food.

**Reason #4: Presence of lesions in the stomach**

Ulcers and stomach lesions developed in rats that were fed with GM tomatoes for a period of 28 days.  More disturbingly, the study found unexplained deaths among 20% of the 40 rats used in the laboratory test.  This particular study was commissioned by the company Calgene, the producer of the GMO tomato called Flavr Savr.

**Reason #5: Aging of the liver**

Another experiment carried out utilized GM soy fed to mice for a period of 2 years. The result showed rapid changes in the hepatocyte metabolism. Moreover, indications of liver aging such as calcium signaling and stress response changes were found. Mice, which were fed with non-GMO soy showed complete normal liver function.

**Reason #6: Dense uterine lining**

For a period of 15 months, female rats were given genetically engineered soy.  At the end of the test period, results show significant thickening in the lining of the uterus. Additionally, the study recorded changes in the ovaries of these mice as compared to those who took non-GMO soy.  The lining of the uterus, also referred to as the epithelium, had higher number of cells.

**Reason #7: Unstable functioning of the pancreas, testes, and liver**

The internal organs of mice fed with GMO soy demonstrated instability, particularly for the pancreas, testes, and liver. After tests were conducted, scientists have found that there was an abnormal formation of nuclei and nucleoli among the liver cells.

## Reason #8:  Presence of toxins in the liver and kidney

There are now 19 different studies showing the effects of GMO soy and Bt Maize in mammals. Among the most disturbing results is the consistent and heavy presence of toxins in the liver and kidneys. Long-term feeding trials are currently under way to validate the chronicity of this condition.

## Reason #9:    Altered gut bacteria formation and blood biochemistry

Using GMO rice for 90 days, rats demonstrated an increased water intake. These GMO rice-fed rats displaced unstable blood biochemistry. Presence of altered bacteria in the gut was observed, which could consequently lead to disturbed digestive system functions and inefficient nutrition absorption.

## Reason #10:  Enlarged liver

Monsanto GM canola was used in another study involving rats. For a period of four weeks, these rats developed enlarged organs, particularly the liver. Abnormal increase in the liver size is a sign of toxicity.

# Chapter 4- Know the 'Big Four'

In order to completely engage in a GMO-free diet, it is important to get acquainted with the biggest companies that produce them. Following is a quick overview of the biggest names in the GMO industry.

**Monsanto**

Now considered as the 'Mother of Agricultural Biotechnology', Monsanto has gained grounds in the field of genetic engineering of seeds of corn, oil seeds, cottons, and vegetables. The company's flagship product is a herbicide called Roundup, which has eventually faced bouts of criticisms from different sectors. Other Monsanto products include Aspartame (artificial sweetener often used in bottled drinks), Agent Orange DEKALB, Recombinant **Bovine Growth Hormone (rBGH)** Seminis seeds, Asgrow, and Deltapine.

**Syngenta**

Established in Basel, Switzerland, Syngenta is considered as one of the biggest GMO-producing companies in the world. It is among the leading biotechnology and agrochemical corporations. The company has significantly contributed to the GMO realm with its controversial product – Atrazine. This product functions as fungicide. Other Syngenta products are genetically modified corn, tomatoes, beans, soybeans, and flowers.

**Dupont**

E. I. Du Pont De Nemours & Company (DuPont) is a biotechnology corporation, which is making waves in the fields of agriculture and chemistry. This company manufactures consumer products in various domains such as communications, electronics, nutrition, transportation, apparel, and constructions. It is now regarded as the third among the biggest chemical makers in the world. One of its five divisions works solely on the production of genetically modified seeds.

## Bayer

Bayer AG is a member company of the Bayer Corporation, which is a major holding company. Aside from biotechnology, the company is also known for its wide range of products in the fields of healthcare, pharmaceutical, agrochemical, and plastics.

# Chapter 5-Practical Tips on Avoiding GMOs

Going natural or organic is still considered the best way to ensure no GMOs are consumed. But many people are still ill at ease with the thought of possibly purchasing an item from the grocery store with GMO-based ingredient. To address this concern, check the following tips that could help you distinguish GMO-based products the next time you hit the supermarket.

**Tip #01**: Be accustomed to Non-GMO Project Seal. There are products on the shelves that bear the logo (see book cover), which are independently verified by a third party in North America. The presence of the seal can reassure that the product underwent independent verification conducted by NonGMOProject.org.

**Tip #02:** At present, labeling is still highly scrutinized by others, thereby making them illegal to use. Instead of looking for a specific 'Non-GMO' label, you can always check labels that say "100% Organic". Another hint is to purchase items with a label that says "Made with Organic Ingredients."

**Tip #03:** Be more vigilant in checking the ingredients. Know that the top GMO crops are canola, sugar, corn, yellow squash, papaya, soy and cottonseeds. Watch out for genetically engineered zucchini. Furthermore, products sold in the North America with sugar ingredients are derived from a combination of GMO and non-GMO. Artificial hormones are indicators of GMOs. For example, if you see rBGH and rBST, then there is a good chance that the food sold is GMO-based.

**Tip #04:** The digital realm and your mobile phone can be your top ally in checking for GMO products. You can find downloadable brochures as well as phone applications, which are designed principally to educate you on GMOs and to help you in your shopping routines.

See the following chapters for the top Apps and list of ingredients you need to familiarize yourself with when aiming for a GMO-free diet.

# Chapter 6- Uncover the Hidden GMOs

Due to political concerns over GMO labeling, products cannot be directly categorized as GMOs. To reduce the risks of consuming GMO-linked products, it is essential to know ingredients, which may contain GMO sources. Next time you go to your supermarket, check your processed food product, if it contains any of the following:

| | | |
|---|---|---|
| Clycodextrin | Canola | Baking Powder |
| Cobalamin | Condensed Milk | soy protein isolate |
| Corn oil | Dextrose | Cornstarch |
| soy flour | barbeque marinade | Diacetyl |
| Equal lecithin | Glutamate | soy milk |
| modified food starch | glycerol monooleate | tocopherols (vit E) |
| hydrogenated starch | leucine | Phenylalanine |
| teriyaki marinades | isoflavones | lactic acid |
| soy oil | sorbitol | malt |
| cider | maltose | malt extract |
| glycerol | modified starch | Glyceride |
| oleic acid | inositol | Citric Acid |

| malitol | Dextrin | soy isolates |
|---------|---------|--------------|
| stearic acid | soy lecithin | tempeh |
| milk powder | tocopherols (vit E) | Glycine |
| hemicellulose | phytic acid | high fructose corn syrup (HFCS) |
| Corn Flour | Corn sugar | inversol |
| Aspartame | Cystein | hydrolyzed vegetable protein |
| Dyglyceride | Erythritol | mannitol |
| mono and diglycerides | Glycerin | milo starch |
| Cellulose | tocopherols (vit E) | tempeh |
| textured vegetable protein | Phenylalanine | glycine |
| Corn syrup | lactic acid | maltodextrin |
| malt syrup | malt | Shoyu |
| threonine | malt extract | Confectioners' Sugar |
| monosodium | Glyceride | soy sauce |

| | | |
|---|---|---|
| glutamate (MSG) | | |
| protein isolate | Citric Acid | invert sugar |
| tamari | soy isolates | whey powder |
| inverse syrup | soy protein | |

The list is extracted from The Institute for Responsible Technology, one of the leading institutions in raising awareness on genetically modified or engineered crops. The group is present in 30 countries and was established in 2003.

# Chapter 7- Apps to Zap your GMO Diet Temptation

Yes, you can also put your fingers to work in ensuring a GMO-free diet for you and your family. Many Non-Government Organizations and other institutions have commissioned developers to help them spread awareness through phone applications. Now, as the battle against GMO presses on, you can do your share by clicking a button or two and download any of these recommended apps. There are 10 apps to choose from, and each has a quick summary to help you handpick (*or maybe finger-pick*) the one that's perfect for you. So click, tap, and zap those GMOs now.

## Buycott

The company is mainly known for standing up for its principles. The name may sound cute, but the advocacy the group supports is not mignon in any way. This particular app can provide you helpful information on how the product is manufactured. It can demonstrate the different companies involved in allowing the product to break into the market. Another interesting feature of this free app is that it has contact information of different companies to which you can send your queries or opinion. In a nutshell, it is an app that educates and communicates.

## GMO Checker

As the name suggests, this app works like a quick 'search' engine allowing you to immediately identify GMO-free products. It makes use of color-coded legends, which will enable you to decode GMO-based ingredients. You can immediately check products, if they are vegan, organic, or gluten-free. The app bears a user-friendly interface and only costs a fraction of a price. For only $3.99, you can download and immediately use this application.

## True Food

If you happen to be the meticulous type of consumer or shopper, then this app is perfect for you. Compared to the other apps, True Food always responds real-time. You can regularly get updates, tips, and news alerts on GMO food products. Moreover, this application is capable of suggesting alternatives so you can maintain a GMO-free diet.

## Non-GMO Project Shopping Guide

The name says it all. This app is your digital guide that allows you to shop smart. The source of this app - Non-GMO Project's Product Verification Program, is an existing institution that collaborates with several other corporations in raising awareness on the adverse effects of GMO products. As most of the apps in this list, this one is free as well.

## ShopNoGMO

This application is intended to be used by shoppers and by those who are fond of dining out. This app is capable of giving you options when shopping and decoding potential GMO-based ingredient on your food when you are at the restaurant. In addition, the application also contains relevant information on how you can source out organic food easily.

## Healthy Food, Allergens, GMOs & Nutrition Scanner

Referred to as 'The Scanner', this app can instantly read labels of the products you are about to purchase from the supermarket. It can decode the additives included in the product and highlight the nutritional value of the food you are about to feed your family. The scanner gives a certain 'rating' so you can immediately recognize how healthful one particular item is. Users, however, need to pay a minimal $3.99 to be able to download this useful app.

## ipiit, The Food Ambassador

The Food Ambassador has massive information within its database that is useful in identifying food products contaminated with GMO-based ingredients. Apart from GMO data, there are now roughly 210,000 relevant pieces of information on Lactose, Gluten, and HFCS. The app is built on a user-friendly interface allowing users to change the settings. Active users are allowed to take part in the on-line community where they can rate food items.

### Fruit Checker

If you love fruit, but are afraid to consume genetically engineered fruit, then you will love this app. The Fruit Checker is capable of tracking data on a particular fruit product and distinguishing those, which are certified organic from the non-organic ones. If you would like to know where a particular fruit was grown, then clicking on one of its button will do the trick. For merely $0.99, you can have this functional app on your device.

### Chemical Maze

Fun as it may sound, but this app has a serious job to do. The Chemical maze is not only useful in identifying the harmful ingredients on your food; it can also immediately check for potential hazardous raw materials in your pet products and cosmetics. The 'basic' app is free for everyone to download. However, the app contains added features, which require a minimal cost on your end. For an app this useful, it is surely worth every single penny you pay for it.

### Barcode and PLU Label Reader

Using barcodes, you can immediately track the main ingredients in your food product. This app requires users to manually key in the barcode for it to extract information about a product. It costs less than $2.00 and has received plenty of positive feedback from users.

If you dread the idea of consuming GMO foods, then download any of these applications. Moreover, you will find brochures or reading materials that are free and downloadable online. In your quest against GMO products, it is essential to take the extra mile in keeping yourself updated.

# Chapter 8 – How to Start Your GMO-free Diet

Take it from the experts. The founding director of The Institute for Responsible Technology, Jeffrey M. Smith, has devoted his career to raising awareness on the potential health risks brought about by GMO-related foods. In his book, "Genetic Roulette: The Gamble of Our Lives", the GMO expert has reiterated the health risks of GMOs including immunity problems, infertility, accelerated aging, disturbance in organ and system functions, and insulin regulation.

So how can you really start a GMO-free diet? There are simple steps you can take, even without having to become an expert on the subject. If you wish to avoid the adverse effects of GMO foods, then you can do so by following the following simple steps:

## Step 01: Stick with ORGANIC crops

Vitamin expert Kathy Gruver has mentioned several times that organic crops have higher level of vitamin and mineral content. Going organic is also highly recommended by the The USDA National Organic Standards. You may not be extremely pleased with the price of these organic commodities, but the bottom line is – you should never put a price tag on health.

## Step 02: Say NO to Aspartame

This can be a tough call for diet sodas enthusiasts, but Aspartame (the artificial sweetener used in calorie-free drinks) is sometimes made from GMOs. This may be a good reason to refrain from carbonated drinks altogether, thus avoiding Aspartame and enjoying a much sweeter and healthier lifestyle.

## Step 03: Say Hello to More Veggies and Fruit

Fresh produce is most of the time non-GMO. However, you may want to avoid the isle where you can find papaya from Hawaii or sweet corn from China. Moreover, try avoiding yellow summer squash and zucchini, if you are not certain where they were grown.

### Step 04: Subtract the additives from your diet

Are you fond of instant or canned food? Do you enjoy loading up on processed food? Well, you may want to think twice next time. Know that the top 5 or commonly used GMOs are corn, cotton, soya, sugar beets, and canola. If you check your food label, these may be disguised as corn syrup, sweetening agent, or thickeners. If you can resist buying them, then that's a good thing. If you can't, then you can try looking for alternatives instead.

### Step 05: Check the label, and then check the seal

The mere fact that GMO-producing companies do not really inform the public which products contain GMOs does not mean you cannot avoid them. You can outsmart these companies by looking for the **"Non-GMO Project Verified seal"** instead. But what does it really mean? This seal signifies that a certain product has undergone a verification process initiated by the Non-GMO Project.

### Step 06: When dining out, take time to call first

There is no harm in asking. Before you dine out next time, you can call ahead to check whether certain dishes are cooked with canola oil. You may also want to ask if they can replace zucchini with another ingredient you are more comfortable with instead. You do not need to ask directly, if the restaurant uses GMO-based products – that would be a tad over-the-top. However, you can ask for their best dishes and evaluate the main ingredients they use.

### Step 07: Load up on fiber

If you are looking for a healthier option, then fiber-rich grains, beans, lentils and nuts are a good choice. Most of these grains are non-GMO, and therefore, are proven safe for consumption.

### Step 08: Impart your knowledge, take part in the **Tipping Point Campaign**

The Tipping Point Campaign is a network of activists who are devoted in educating small communities on risks of GMO. The goal is to gain people's commitment in avoiding GMO-based products so that the manufacturers or producers will be forced to eradicate them from the market.

You cannot truly alter your diet in one go. However, you can start altering it by educating yourself on the danger of GMO-based food. Your health is unquestionably the most important aspect of your existence. Reducing your exposure to this food will inevitably aid you in building healthier and better eating habits.

# Chapter 9 – Kids and GMOs

Children thrive on nutrition and parents would do just about anything to ensure that children get the nutrition they really need. However, the reality is that many of the food products patronized by children may contain GMOs – cookies, snack bars, cereals, crackers, and other processed items. It is a sad fact that in the US, roughly 80% of the food may be linked to GMO-based ingredients.

Several studies have shown that GMO-based products pose great risks on an average person. But what about kids? These small and more vulnerable beings are easy targets of allergens and other health hazards.

Here are reasons why it is NEVER a good idea to serve GMO foods to your little ones:

**Reason # 01**: Children have a much more vulnerable immune systems making them highly susceptible to different allergies

Children below 10 years of age are generally four times more susceptible to allergies than the average adults. Moreover, those who are below the age 2 are prone to the greater risks. These children often develop allergies to food that contains allergens, a characteristic common to GMO-based products. GM corn or Bt Maize in particular is a problem for kids, especially those who are corn-dependent for their protein. In the UK, for instance, there has been a significant increase in allergies due to consumption of BT corn-based products particularly in baby food.

**Reason # 02:** Children who consume GM products are at risk of contracting antibiotic resistant illnesses

Ear infections are far more common in kids, than in adults. Kids who are used to having GM products often encounter strains of bacteria that are highly antibiotic-resistant. Due to this medical condition, The British Medical Association is now working on a moratorium of these GM-based foods.

**Reason # 03**: GMOs impact the development pace of young bodies

Most of the studies on the impact of GMOs used adult mice in their laboratory experiments. These mice have shown damage in organs in as early as one week after the commencement of the experiments. Damages recorded include smaller brain developed, disturbed immune systems, liver atrophy, and the presence of cancerous cells in the intestine. Moreover, it is safe to conclude that such impact could trigger more easily in small human bodies.

**Reason # 04:** Children are prone to nutritional issues

As per the 2002 report released by UK's Royal Society, genetic engineering could result to a range of unforeseen adverse changes in the nutritional status of food. With this conclusion came a recommendation stating that parents should conduct rigorous research before deciding on preparing GM-based foods for children. The same recommendation was given to the elderly and to those with chronic diseases. Two of the potential side effects of altered nutritional state mentioned were on the sexual development of babies and bowel obstruction when fed with GM soy-based infant formula.

**Reason # 05**: Babies and young children may have problems with dairy and milk

Dairy products and milk from genetically engineered bovine growth hormone (rbGH) - treated cows contain a higher amount of hormone IGF-1. This hormone is one of the leading contributors to prostate and breast cancer cell development.

At present, there are medical and research institutions calling for more studies to determine whether IGF-1 is safe for children and babies. Among these institution is the Council on Scientific Affairs of the American Medical Association. The Cancer Prevention Coalition Chairman has expressed concern on the potential effect of the ingested IGF-1 hormone. He has reiterated his concern over the possible allergic and hormonal effects of rbGH when absorbed by the blood of children. In addition, he also highlighted that cow hormones have the potential to produce adrenaline-type chemicals, which function like steroids. These effects normally lead to serious medical heart problems. Children who consume these products are likely to develop serious medical conditions when they get older.

It is crucial for parents from all walks of life to take part in the crusade against GMO foods. If your family has already been used to consuming products with GMO-based ingredients, know that it is never too late to make that change. Companies, Non-Government Organizations, and Research Institutions from all around the world have been working rigorously and spending millions of dollars to ensure that consumers are protected from the health risks posed by GMO foods. You, too, can help in protecting your own family. Making wise decisions when shopping for food, reading news alerts on the subject, or e-mailing your questions are among the first measures you can take. Your family only deserves the healthiest of food, and the healthiest of communities. It is time to switch to a diet that is truly, and verified GMO-free!

# Conclusion

Thank you again for downloading this book!

I hope this book was able to help you to fully grasp the importance of consuming non-GMO foods. In the end, it will always be up to YOU- and your willingness to change your habits for the best.

The next step is to start going through your shopping list again, so you can begin embodying this whole new lifestyle. Your family will soon benefit from all these changes, so let me congratulate you in advance.

Finally, if you enjoyed reading this book, I would greatly appreciate your book review on Amazon.com.


Thank you and good luck!

# Preview Of 'Juicing for Health: The Essential Guide To Healing Common Diseases with Proven Juicing Recipes and Staying Healthy For Life' by Donna Cavanaugh

## *Acne*

### Lemon Twist (morning drink)
**Ingredients**
- 1 Lemon
- 1 cup hot water

### Carrot Clear
**Ingredients**
- 8 Carrots
- 2 stalks Celery
- ½ cup Watercress

### Dandelion Leaves Juice
**Ingredients**
- 1 handful Dandelion leaves
- 1 Apple
- 1 Red Beet
- 1 Lemon

**Explanation**

Acne is an inflammatory disease of the sebaceous glands and hair follicles of the skin that is marked by the eruption of pimples or pustules, especially on the face. Fresh lemon, dandelion, carrots, celery, beets and apples purify the blood, removing metabolic waste and changing pH from acidic to alkaline

# *Allergies*

## Red Velvet
**Ingredients**
- 4 Carrots
- 2 stalks Celery
- 1 cup Pineapple
- 1 thumb Ginger
- ½ Red Beet

## Green Beast
**Ingredients**
- 2 Apples
- 3 stalks Celery
- 1 Cucumber
- 1 thumb Ginger
- ½ Lemon (with rind)
- 1 Lime (with rind)
- 1 bunch Parsley
- 2 cups Spinach

**Explanation**

Allergies are triggered where the responses to allergens that your body absorbs from the environment or from your diet, causing heightened immune system responses, usually with inappropriate levels of inflammation or irritation. Pineapple contains the enzyme bromelain, which is widely used by German physicians to treat inflammation and swelling of the nose, ear, and sinuses. Recent scientific research has proven that ginger can be used for therapies of various illnesses due to its antioxidant effects, its ability to inhibit the formation of inflammatory compounds, and its anti-inflammatory effects.

# *Anemia*

## Beet Anemia
### Ingredients
- 4 Carrots
- 2 stalks Celery
- 2 Red Beets
- 1 handful Blackberries
- 2 oz Lettuce

## Explanation
Anemia is a condition where the number of red blood cells or concentrations of hemoglobin are low. Iron is the foundation for hemoglobin, the molecule which is responsible for the transport of oxygen. In Europe, beet juice has been used for centuries as a treatment for anemia, due to its high content of iron, folic acid, Vitamin B1, B2, B6, and vitamins A & C.

Please visit Amazon.com to purchase your copy of Juicing for Health: The Essential Guide To Healing Common Diseases with Proven Juicing Recipes and Staying Healthy For Life

www.ingramcontent.com/pod-product-compliance
Lightning Source LLC
Chambersburg PA
CBHW071343310526
45790CB00018B/1266